How to Lose Belly Fat:

A Complete Guide to Losing Weight and Achieving a Flat Belly

© Copyright 2018 by Charlie Mason - All rights reserved.

The following Book is reproduced below with the goal of providing information that is as accurate and reliable as possible. Regardless, purchasing this Book can be seen as consent to the fact that both the publisher and the author of this book are in no way experts on the topics discussed within and that any recommendations or suggestions that are made herein are for entertainment purposes only. Professionals should be consulted as needed prior to undertaking any of the action endorsed herein.

This declaration is deemed fair and valid by both the American Bar Association and the Committee of Publishers Association and is legally binding throughout the United States.

Furthermore, the transmission, duplication or reproduction of any of the following work including specific information will be considered an illegal act irrespective of if it is done electronically or in print. This extends to creating a secondary or tertiary copy of the work or a recorded copy and is only allowed with an express written consent from the Publisher. All additional rights reserved.

The information in the following pages is broadly considered to be a truthful and accurate account of facts and as such any inattention, use or misuse of the information in question by the reader will render any resulting actions solely under their purview. There are no scenarios in which the publisher or the original author of this work can be in any fashion deemed liable for any hardship or damages that may befall them after undertaking information described herein.

Additionally, the information in the following pages is intended only for informational purposes and should thus be thought of as universal. As befitting its nature, it is presented without assurance regarding its prolonged validity or interim quality. Trademarks that are mentioned are done without written consent and in no way be considered an endorsement from the trademark holder.

Table of Contents

BONUS: 6
Introduction 7
Chapter 1: Welcome 8
    Understanding the Biological Process 11
    What is the Difference Between Calories and Fat? 11
Chapter 3: Understanding Energy Consumption in the Body . 18
    Understanding Energy 18
Chapter 4: How Your Body Changes 22
    Your Changing Anatomy 22
Chapter 5: What NOT to Eat 26
    Why a Healthy Diet Matters 26
    Wisdom to Consider 31
Chapter 6: Healthy Diet 33
    Diets to Consider 33
    Foods to Eat 33
    How Much You Should Eat 34
Chapter 7: Meal Prep 37
    Baked Honey-Mustard Chicken 37
    Slow Cooker Pork Tenderloin 38
    Roasted Vegetables 39
    Fish Tacos 40
    Lentil Soup 42
    Turkey Veggie Meatloaf Cups 43
    Grandma's Chicken Noodle Soup 44
    Chicken and Asparagus Pasta 45
    Greek Chicken Pasta 46

Black Bean Chili 47
Feta and Spinach Pita Bake.. 48
Zucchini and Potato Bake... 49
Quinoa Tabbouleh 50
Chapter 8: What to Drink 51
How Can Beverages Help You Lose Weight? 51
Chapter 9: Working with Your Metabolism 55
What is Metabolism?... 55
Chapter 10: Cardio and Strength Training 62
Understanding Exercise 62
What to Watch out For 65
Chapter 11: The Big Picture 66
Conclusion 68
BONUS: 69

BONUS:

As a way of saying thank you for purchasing my book, please use your link below to claim your 3 FREE Cookbooks on Health, Fitness & Dieting Instantly

https://bit.ly/2LEQVu2

You can also share your link with your friends and families whom you think that can benefit from the cookbooks or you can forward them the link as a gift!

Introduction

Congratulations on purchasing the *How to Lose Belly Fat: A Complete Guide to Losing Weight and Achieving a Flat Belly* and thank you for doing so.

The following chapters will discuss the best practices needed to lose weight, get fit, and live a healthier lifestyle. There are no gimmicks here. With hard work and determination, you can have a flat stomach before you know it!

There are plenty of books on this subject on the market, thanks again for choosing this one! Every effort was made to ensure it is full of as much useful information as possible, please enjoy!

Chapter 1: Welcome

Everyone has something about their physique that they want to change. Only 8% of Americans feel content about their physical selves, so keep in mind that you are not alone on this journey to a skinnier you. In fact, in the US more than 50% of men and 70% of women between the ages of 50 and 79 suffer from a condition known as "abdominal obesity". Regardless of your age, weight gain has become an epidemic in the 21st century. This is due to the fact that we are surrounded by high fat, processed food that is readily available to us anytime day or night. As busy adults, it can be hard to focus on some of the most important aspects of our lives, like our health. It is easy to get caught up in everyday priorities. Then we forget what it takes to achieve and maintain a healthy diet and exercise regimen. This is especially true when dealing with belly fat. It can be difficult to combat the temptation of convenient, tasty food but with the right mindset, anything is possible.

As we know, any unwanted fat is seen as an obstacle, but belly fat can be especially difficult to get rid of. Belly fat can be more than just an unsightly annoyance, though. It is also incredibly bad for your health. Belly fat, also referred to as visceral fat, is a big risk factor for stroke, type 2 diabetes, heart disease, and high blood pressure. Visceral fat refers to the fat that builds up deep underneath your skin. It sits right on top of your abdominal muscles, making it difficult to feel or see them. Most health organizations use BMI (Body Mass Index) to predict the risk of fat-related illnesses and determine your weight. You can calculate your BMI in two different ways. You can find calculators to determine your BMI online, or you can divide your weight in kilograms by your height in meters squared. A BMI of 27.3 is considered overweight for women, and a BMI of 27.8 is considered overweight for men. Do not let the numbers intimidate you. Regardless of your BMI, you have taken the right step to have a fabulously trim abdomen and a healthier lifestyle.

It is easy to believe that belly fat is the most stubborn fat to defeat. This is something that most of us have known for years, but why is it so hard to get off and keep off? Scientists claim that belly fat is more difficult to shift than any other part of the body. This is because fat cells in the abdomen do not respond as quickly to the fat burning process known as lipolysis. Combine this with a busy schedule and an infinite amount of unhealthy options, and you have stubborn belly flab that seems impossible to lose.

Of course, dieting isn't the only component of kicking the flab. Exercise plays a huge role in burning fat and building muscle. Regardless of what you see online, doing 100 sit-ups a day will not give you a flat stomach. Not even those state of the art abdominal machines that you see on late night infomercials will give you the results you're looking for without help. Truthfully, the combination of consistent diet and exercise is the only way you will achieve the rock hard body that you have been envisioning for years. Just remember that diet and exercise do not have to be boring. Find an activity that you enjoy and foods that you love to make the transition that much easier. Even recruiting a friend to accompany you on the journey can turn a chore into a great time! Lucky for you, this guild will provide you with all of the knowledge needed to be successful with your new diet and exercise routine.

Now, I know what you are thinking. We have all seen those diets that claim to be the miracle solution to your weight loss problems. They typically involve unorthodox methods such as the liquid diet or the "Crazy for Cabbage" diet. Even though there are hundreds, upon hundreds of fad diets circulating the media that claim to make you skinny overnight, you always end up disappointed and hungry. Unfortunately, there is no magic solution to losing belly fat hidden in this book. Like most things, the reward of your perfect body will come from hard work and consistency. Tackling this lifestyle change won't be a walk in the park, but the hardest part is making the decision to take the first step. Take a moment to congratulate yourself for committing to a more fit, happier you!

Regardless of your experience level with diet and exercise, *How to Lose Belly Fat: A Complete Guide to Losing Weight and Achieving a Flat Belly* will teach you the fundamentals of shedding excess weight and keeping it off. Whether you're trying to get that sexy figure back or to lose weight to fit into the perfect dress for a special occasion, this guide will give you the information you need to achieve your goals and look fantastic while doing it! As you move through the book, you will see that we have broken down the components of a healthy lifestyle geared towards eliminating visceral fat. We have reduced it down to simple, easy to follow sections that will keep you motivated and engaged. You will learn the fundamentals behind fat and calories, how your metabolism works, and how to work with it, the right kind of exercise and diet needed to create and maintain your flat belly, what NOT to eat, and physical changes to expect as you transition into your new body.

If you are ready to get a flat stomach, learn about foods that fuel you, look amazing in anything, and become a more confident person then hold on for the ride! This guide will teach you a natural approach to fat loss and will have you turning heads in no time!

Chapter 2: Understanding Belly Fat and Calories

Understanding the Biological Process

Ecologically, our bodies were designed for survival. Thousands of years ago when we hunted and scavenged for food, having extra fat reserves was critical for living a long life. Now that we have restaurants on every corner, the mechanisms once designed to keep up alive are now doing the opposite. Humans are hardwired to love sugar and fat. This is because sugar and fats were once utilized as lightweight energy provisions that kept our ancestors alive. Fat and sugars weigh less than muscle, so our instincts tell us to take every opportunity to gorge on fatty, sugary foods to avoid starving to death. This is also why sugar and fats taste so good. Now we have a digestive tract that is geared towards storing as many excess calories as possible, which is unfortunate in a society where almost everything is calorie dense. Even though our bodies are made to hold onto excess weight, like belly fat, that does not mean that we can't fight back.

What is the Difference Between Calories and Fat?

The first step to understanding weight loss is recognizing the difference between fat and calories. Fats are essential for human life. It is one of the six nutrients required to have a healthy body and mind along with carbohydrates, proteins, water, vitamins, and minerals. Three of the six essential nutrients provide the body with calories. Those are proteins, carbohydrates, and fats. Calories are units of measurement categorized as the amount of energy that is released when our body processes food. The body stores excess calories in fat cells, of which we have an infinite number. The higher the calorie count, the more energy that food can provide for our body. When we consume more calories than we need, our body stores them as fat.

Understanding Fat

Fat has a multitude of function within the human body. Fat can be stored in places other than the abdominal area, such as the liver and skeletal muscle. Fat is responsible for regulating hormone production, helping transport vitamins and minerals around the body, providing cell structure, and protecting vital organs. It serves as a source of energy for the infinitude of cell function and is even responsible for approximately 70% of the energy used for bodily function while at rest. Needless to say, we cannot survive without fat nutrients.

Different Types of Fat

You may have seen or heard the words "saturated" or "trans fat" throughout your lifetime, but what do they actually mean? Trans fats are fats produced from oil that is created through a food processing method called partial hydrogenation. You can find these types of fats in all processed food such as fast food. These fats have the tendency to lower good cholesterol levels or high-density lipoprotein (HDL) and raise bad cholesterol levels or low-density lipoprotein (LDL). Having high cholesterol is directly linked with heart disease and of course, weight gain.

Unfortunately, many of the foods that we find delicious contain saturated fat. They are calorie rich with little to no nutritional value. Examples of these foods include bacon, sausage, potatoes chips, and hamburgers. Protein sources, especially dairy products, and red meat contain saturated fats. It is important to understand what kind of protein will benefit your weight loss as opposed to which kind can hinder your progress. To achieve a flat belly you should get your protein from lean meats or vegetables and legumes such as beans, lentils, and tofu.

Even though fat is one of three essential nutrients that provide us with energy; it has over twice as many calories per gram than both of its counterparts. A gram of carbohydrates or protein would render around 4 calories, while a gram of fat contains 9 calories. Basically, you can eat the same amount of carbs or protein for half of the calories of fat. The simple explanation to achieving your weight loss goals might be to only eat food that is low in fat, and while eating less fatty foods will help you shed pounds, it is not enough. Even if you eat low calorie, non-fat foods, excess calories can still be hoarded away for the winder, especially in your belly. You have to pay close attention to how many calories you consume from all three types of nutrients a day. To lose weight, you need to have a caloric deficit, which you can achieve by burning more calories than you consume.

Not all kinds of fat are bad for you. Unsaturated fats come from vegetable oils, nuts, and seeds. Unsaturated and monounsaturated fats aid in boosting good cholesterol levels, and at the same time, decreasing bad cholesterol levels. They provide key nutrients that allow cells to absorb fat-soluble vitamins such as vitamin D. Polyunsaturated fats are also a healthy alternative to saturate and trans fats. Omega-3 and Omega-6 are some of the Polyunsaturated fats, which are paramount for regulating blood pressure. You should replace your daily intake of saturated fats with unsaturated fats like monounsaturated and polyunsaturated nutriments. You can find these nutrients in avocados, nuts, seeds, fatty fish, and tofu.

How to Determine How Much Fat You Are Eating

Read labels, and then read them again. The amount of fat will be listed on the nutrition facts on the back of the product you want to purchase. The total calories will be listed, as well as the total calories from fat. Most food labels also list the daily percentage of fat within each serving. Choose foods with a low percentage of daily fat. The amount of fat you need to consume per day varies on how many calories you consume per day.

Your Daily Calorie Intake	Fat You Should Consume Daily
2,500	83 grams
2,200	73 grams
2,000	65 grams
1,800	60 grams
1,200	40 grams

Reading labels can be tedious and confusing, especially when the print on the label is meant to fool you. You may see some products sporting a "low-fat" or "low cholesterol" label. Manufacturers have to meet government regulations to use these labels on their food. If a product says fat or sugar-free, it actually means that it has less than 0.5 grams of sugar or fat. If the label says "low fat" it contains 3 grams of fat or less. Keep that in mind as you shop in order to avoid unhealthy fats that directly keep you from burning fat.

Stress and Fat

Like most aspects of the human body, fat is affected by stress. It is important to monitor your stress levels and recognize what brings you tension in optimize weight loss. When your body endures a stressful moment, your flight or fight reflexes are triggered. This causes your cortisol levels (the stress hormo[ne] to skyrocket, all the while increasing insulin levels, and lowering your blood sugar. This results in hunger. Your body assumes that you have used up a large number of calories during your reaction to the stress, such as fleeing the dangerous situation or choosing to fight. Even though there has been no rigorous physical activity, your brain tricks your body into thinking that you need to replenish the lost calories, causing you to overeat. These are the times that you find yourself searching out a slice of pizza or fried chicken. They call this type of food comforting for a reason. The brain releases chemicals that create a calming sensation while ingesting this food, which correlates back to our prehistorically need for fats and sugars to keep us alive.

Understanding Calories

Calories are units of measurement categorized as the amount of energy that is released when our body breaks down and digests food. They are in everything you eat from gum, to ketchup, to mints, and even vitamins. Just like fats, not all calories are created equally. Some calories are considered "empty" meaning that they have no nutritional value whatsoever. Technically, you receive the same amount of energy from empty calories as you do nutrient-rich calories. For example, you could eat 1500 calories of fast food or 1500 calories of vegetables and retain the same amount of energy from both. The difference is that if you ate 1500 calories of fast food, your body would assume that you are using your entire day's energy in that one moment, instead of evenly spreading out your daily caloric intake. This causes you to feel groggy and hungry long before your workday is over. Eating empty calories can lead to a never-ending cycle of feeling famished and overeating.

How Calories Affect Fat

In the age of calorie counting and fad diets, it is easy to believe that the fewer calories you consume, the better. This is not the case since everyone has a minimal level of calories that one should consume per day. The number varies depending on your BMI, age, activity level, and gender. One pound of fat is equivalent to 3,500 calories. That's how many calories you need to burn to lose that much fat and decrease your caloric intake by 500 to lose a pound a week. Keep in mind that as you lose weight your caloric need will decrease.

Since calories are basically your body's fuel, it is important that you have enough to maintain your energy throughout your waking hours. Knowing the number of calories you need to eat in order to lose weight is the key in the process of getting your flat belly. You should also be conscious of what types of calories you are eating, since eating empty calories will cause you to be hungry and more likely to stray from your diet.

How Calories Affect Muscle Mass

When it comes to building muscle the type of calories you are consuming is very important. If you were to eat 200 calories of ice cream, it would be absorbed into the body very differently than if you ate 200 calories of chickpeas. Since chickpeas are nutrient rich and high in fiber, it is likely that 10% of those calories won't be absorbed at all. You are much more likely to gain muscle mass when eating a diet that is high in protein and nutrient-rich opposed to a diet that is nutrient-poor and low in fiber.

How to Determine How Many Calories You Are Eating

To find the number of calories in a product and the number of calories from fat, find the nutrition facts on the back of the product. It is common knowledge that the Food and Drug Administration (FDA) regulates all caloric calculations from every food supplier on the market. What the FDA doesn't want you to know is that they could not possibly double-check everyone's caloric calculations down to the decimal, to the point that a product is not considered "mislabeled" unless it is more than 20% off. This means that not every calorie count listed is correct. If you pick something up that seems too healthy to be true, go for something more reliable, such as larger brands or plant-based, whole foods.

Exercise and Calories

As previously mentioned, exercise plays a huge part in getting rid of that flat tire around your middle and toning the muscles underneath it to give you that sexy figure. How do calories and exercise inter-relate? As you know, calories are units of measurement designed to determine energy within the human body. The more energy you use, the more calories you burn. Getting out and moving around will get rid of those extra calories. All exercises affect your muscle mass, whether it is walking, running, biking, or swimming. This allows your body to continuously burn calories long after your workout is over. Once you begin to burn more calories you consume, you begin to lose weight.

Chapter 3: Understanding Energy Consumption in the Body

Understanding Energy

The topic of energy is a hot one in the 21st century. Scientists are constantly trying to find a bigger and better source of energy to power the world. Think of your body like a fine-tuned machine that needs energy (food) to function properly. You can utilize the way your body consumes vitality to help you get fit and healthy!

In science class, we were taught that energy cannot be created nor destroyed. This is a fundamental law of science that will forever be true, but what does it mean when we say "burning calories"? Basically, it just means burning the units of power needed to make you go. Energy cannot be destroyed, but it must be converted from one form to another such as mechanical energy to help us move, thermal energy to keep us warm, and electrical energy that allows us to use our brain. The type of energy used within the body is called adenosine triphosphate (ATP). ATP is technically chemical reaction that our body uses to carry out our biological processes. Carbs, fats, and proteins are the nutrients that provide us with strength, but fats provide the most power. These functions aid in hormone regulation, blood circulation, digestion, and cell growth. If some calories are not immediately used as energy, they are stored as fat.

Types of Energy

Depending on what you eat, calories can be broken down into different types of energy that your body will use immediately or save for later. For example, if you eat a meal rich in carbohydrates and poor in whole grain, these calories are quickly reduced down to glucose, which is used to power your muscles. This will cause your blood sugar to rise, and shortly after, your energy levels to fall. Eating a meal rich in whole grains will allow your body to move through the digestion process much slower, allowing you energy reserves to be consistent throughout the day. You want to fuel your body in order to burn fat around your middle and build muscle. Keep this in mind as you implement your new exercise regimen!

How Diet Affects Your Energy

Now that you understand how energy affects the body, you can begin to plan your dietary needs around the amount of energy you will need to become a slimmer you! To achieve optimal amounts of power, you will need to eat a balanced diet that is rich in vegetables, healthy fats, healthy oils, unrefined carbohydrates, and proteins. Even though sweets, candies, and energy drinks can give you a boost of hyperactivity, you want to stay away from them in order to avoid the crash they provide a few hours after consumption. Another way to keep your energy levels up would be to eat frequently throughout your day. Consistent healthy snacking could replace the basic three-meals-a-day rule. Your brain needs constant nutrients to function, so when you munch on fruits or veggies every few hours, you are more likely to feel energized and have a higher cognitive function.

Make Caffeine Your Friend

Caffeine is such a huge part of American culture. We glamorize a busy schedule and effectively cramming everything that we need to get done into an 8-hour workday, so of course, we love caffeine! Most people wake up to a coffee first thing in the morning and feel that they are unable to function without it. Caffeine is a stimulant, so it has the ability to increase your energy levels. Depending on how much you consume and when, caffeine can be a helpful resource for making you more alert, but be careful. Consuming too much caffeine can cause serious jitters and even insomnia. So, enjoy it in moderation before the busiest time of your day. Also, watch out for energy drinks and sodas. They are high in sugar and will result in a downward spiral that will leave you feeling tired and hungry.

Fat and Energy

If you suffer from being overweight like 30% of the American population, you probably spend a good chunk of your time being fatigued. This is because the extra weight on your body, especially around your midsection, puts extra pressure on your joints. This makes physical activity difficult and puts you at risk for arthritis, sleep apnea, and asthma. Your body uses a large amount of energy when combatting pain and this can cause you to feel tired. When you carry around a fat belly, it puts more pressure on your lungs and heart, causing you to be even more exhausted. Controlling and maintaining your weight can help you regain your energy and reduce health risks. Reducing your weight has also been linked to a reduction in depression. Depression zaps your energy and prohibits you from finding the motivation needed to live a healthy lifestyle. Not only will getting healthy give you a flatter belly and more energy, but it will also make you a happier person! If exercise does not improve your depression, consider talking with your doctor.

Stress and Energy

Stress reduction goes an incredibly long way when it comes to burning fat and working for that flat belly. The more stress you encounter, the more cortisol your body produces. The stress hormone causes you to be hungry and tired. When you give in to the cravings, the calories go straight to your belly, hips, and thighs. Reducing your stress levels can sound difficult and possibly intimidating, but once you begin a routine of relaxation practices, you find that your energy increases and your overall body functions have improved. Meditation is a popular practice all over the world that has been known to reduce stress levels. Some people use exercise as a form of moving meditation, but there are countless other ways to live a stress-free life. As you begin to implement a healthy diet and exercise into your life, be sure to incorporate relaxation strategies as well. After all, becoming the person you want to be should be a positive experience, not a stressful one.

Chapter 4: How Your Body Changes

Your Changing Anatomy

Now that you understand calories, fat, and energy, it is time to prepare for the changes you will go through once you implement a healthy diet and exercise routine. The basics of weight loss tell us that if we consume fewer calories, our caloric needs will shrink and so will our body. It sounds simple, but there are countless aspects of weight loss to consider. Once you get into the swing of your new fitness routine, you may not be able to feel or see yourself shrinking because weight loss begins on a molecular level. As you eat healthily and work out, your fat cells begin to shrink. The fat that has been stored in your fat cells is finally able to fulfill its purpose as energy that will be used by your body for power. The fat that was once hanging around your belly has now been broken down into its final elements, which are carbon dioxide and water. Most of the fat that you lose will leave the body through your respiratory system. That's right. You are breathing the fat out of your body. The fat that doesn't evacuate through your nostrils will leave the body through sweat, urine, and other bodily fluids.

Unfortunately, your fat cells remain where they are. Remember when we talked about having an infinite amount of fat cells? As humans, our bodies are engineered to fear the worst, such as starving to death. So, we have to trick our bodies with diet and exercise to prevent those fat cells from filling up again.

Water Weight

Our bodies accumulate water naturally, but eating clean will allow you to flush the water relatively quickly. You will lose fat, but first, you will lose water weight. Regardless of what kind of diet you choose to do, the water weight will always be the first thing to come off of your body. Losing water is actually what gives you a substantial amount of weight loss right after you begin your new lifestyle. After you have shed all of the water, the number on the scale tends to plateau. Do not let this kill your motivation, though. Getting rid of the water weight is the first step to losing belly fat. Once the water is gone, your body begins the process of burning your fat reservoirs, like the one in your middle.

Challenges *to* Expect

Keep in mind that with any weight loss experience, you are constantly fighting against your body. Your body biologically does not want you to lose weight because it thinks you need fat to survive in case you are ever deprived of food. Your body will notice that you are eating less and release chemicals that make you feel hungry. To combat this, eat plenty of fibrous and protein filled foods to keep you fueled. Along with water weight and fat, you are also losing muscle tissue, which is the opposite of what you want to do. Keeping up with your exercise routine is crucial to achieving a flat belly and a healthy lifestyle.

Positives to Look Forward To

As you go through this process, you may feel like your body has a mind of its own. Adjusting to your new lifestyle won't be completely bad, though. There are a number of positive side effects to look forward to. First and foremost, you are going to feel better. Your new diet should provide you with enough energy to sustain your workout routine, which should also make you feel more energized. Say goodbye to that constant feeling of exhaustion. Once your body is free of the extra pounds, your oxygen intake will be more efficient, making climbing the stairs that much easier to do without losing your breath.

You may find that you remember things better. Studies show that individuals who have implemented a weight loss plan tend to recall information better than those who kept their unhealthy habits. This is due to the fact that when you live a healthier lifestyle, your brain uses more energy to creating memories and less energy when retrieving them, causing your memory function to skyrocket.

You risk of cancer and other weight-related illnesses will lower. This is because your body does not have to waste energy on simple things such as getting around or being tired. With all of this extra time and vitality, your body puts more effort into making sure your cells are healthy and that your systems are functioning properly.

Food may begin to taste different. Some studies show that after individuals lost a significant amount of weight, foods they once enjoyed, such as fast food or highly processed foods, began to taste dull and stale. This caused them to gravitate towards fresh foods that fueled their energy and kept them on track.

You may sleep better. It is common knowledge that a healthy diet and exercise plan can cause you to have a more restful sleep. Since your weight is reducing, especially in the belly area, you will see a significant change in your sleep quality. Even more so if you suffer from sleep disorders such as daytime fatigue, insomnia, or sleep apnea. You might also find that you no longer snore, which creates a better sleeping environment for you and your partner.

You will be happier. Meeting a goal of any kind is cause for celebration, but once you hit your health and fitness goal, you may find that you are the happiest you've ever been. There is a big correlation between a healthy body and a happy mind. With more energy from your diet and more confidence from your slimming waistline, it may be impossible to get the smile off of your face. In fact, scientists have linked weight loss with a reduction of depression. Unfortunately, losing weight isn't a fix-all. 10% of individuals who were depressed before they lost weight were just as depressed after they lost 100 pounds. This is due to underlying causes that should be addressed with your doctor.

Chapter 5: What NOT to Eat

Why a Healthy Diet Matters

Now that you know what you have to look forward to, let's get down to business and determine what you should eliminate from your diet. Even with a detailed exercise routine, eating unhealthy foods will keep you from reaching your flat belly goal. The rule of thumb states that 20% of the washboard abs you dream of are being created in the gym, while the other 80% are made in the kitchen. You would be surprised at how much of an impact unhealthy foods have on your middle. You will find that your new diet gets easier with time. It takes 21 days to start a habit and 21 days to break a habit. You can kill two birds with one stone by committing to clean eating for three weeks. After those three weeks are over, you will find that your healthy lifestyle has taken root. Staying away from foods that cause weight gain may seem difficult at first, but once you begin to see results, nothing will stop you!

Trans Fats

You are most likely familiar with trans fat. It wasn't very long ago that the media ousted trans fats for what they really are: unhealthy. The government even passed a bill deeming trans fat as unsafe to use in food. In a perfect world, all of our food would be trans-fat-free today, but unfortunately, that is not the case. Since this epidemic was so widespread, it will take more than two years for all foods to be free of this substance. Trans fat likes to set up shop in your belly and within your blood vessels. It is important to pay attention to what your food labels say because you never know what you might get. Trans fats are manufactured by injecting hydrogen into unsaturated fats such as vegetable oil. Trans fats have a nasty habit of lowering good cholesterol levels and raising bad cholesterol levels, leading to a risk of heart attack, stroke, inflammation, and insulin resistance. This type of fat can be found in most packaged foods such as potato chips, crackers, cookies, cakes, fast food, along with margarine and spreads. Red meat also contains natural trans fats that are produced when the bacteria in animals' stomachs digest grass; so remember to stick with lean protein sources such as skinless chicken and fish. It is important to read labels when purchasing processed food or avoid it all together. You can swap out your favorite trans fat filled food for unprocessed, plant-based options instead.

Alcohol

Almost everyone takes the opportunity to indulge in a drink after work or in the face of an obligatory social engagement, but did you know that the occasional beer could be the reason that your gut won't budge? Alcohol can have health benefits in tiny amounts, like when you are suffering from a cold, but consuming too much alcohol could have adverse effects on your weight loss. Alcohol is one of the leading factors that contribute to belly fat. Observational studies suggest that consuming more alcohol than needed leads to an increase in excess weight around the abdomen. This phenomenon is also known as "beer gut". Not to mention the fact that alcohol dehydrates your body, making you feel sluggish and hungry. You do not have to abstain from alcohol completely, but cutting back on your intake will significantly reduce your waistline.

Dairy Products

It is overwhelming to think about the number of the products we eat that contain dairy. We cook with it, put it in our cereal, and even our morning coffee. It's crazy to imagine what life would be like without dairy, but over 70% of Americans are lactose intolerant. Lactose intolerance basically means that you do not have the enzyme needed to break down and digest lactose. This leads to bloating, gas, and an upset stomach. Lactose intolerance can be mild to severe. Since it causes the build-up of natural gasses in the stomach, you are much more likely to feel and look bloated. If you suspect that you may be lactose intolerant, try cutting out dairy for a week and see if you notice any changes. Always consult with your doctor before a major diet shift. If you are not lactose intolerant, you will want to avoid dairy products that claim to be "nonfat" or "low-fat". The processing method used to make these products appear healthier but actually removes the healthy fats and replaces it with sugar and sodium. Remember, your body needs healthy fat to survive. You want to eliminate unhealthy, processed fats to attain your flat belly. You can do this by choosing healthier dairy options such as cottage cheese and Greek yogurt.

Soda and Soft Drinks

There is nothing more refreshing than an ice-cold coca cola in the heat of the summer... Except for the perfect body. Soda is everywhere we look from our grocery stores to McDonald's. It is hard to say no to this sweet treat, but the consumption of soda is another leading cause of belly fat. Soda is filled with sugar and empty calories that contribute to excess weight. Studies show that consuming nothing but soda led to the build-up of visceral fat within your midsection. Your body struggles to burn this sugar off, so instead, it is stored in your fat cells. It is reasonable to assume that diet sodas would be a better alternative. The word "diet" is right in the name and it contains 0 calories, but the truth is that these sodas are loaded with artificial sweeteners such as aspartame, saccharin, sucralose, or an herbal sweetener like Stevia. These can be more than five times sweeter than sugar. So do not be fooled into thinking that there is a healthier soda option on the market. Always read the labels on any packaged food or beverage that you buy to ensure that you know what you are consuming. Cutting out soda has an array of health benefits such as strengthening your teeth, lowering your blood sugar, and flattening your belly.

Processed Baked Goods

We are all guilty of walking into the supermarket or gas station only to be tempted by the yummy, packaged baked goods that are scattered around the isles. The unfortunate truth is that dessert cakes, mini donuts, and muffins are packed with sugar and calories. Combine that with virtually no fiber, and you have a contributor to belly fat. This goes for the "freshly baked goods" and Little Debbie cakes at grocery stores, too. Not only are they filled with unwanted sugars; they also contain preservatives that enable them to have a longer shelf life. They could literally be sitting on the shelf for months before anyone decides to pick them up. Can you imagine how long they stick around in your body? Do yourself a favor next time you are craving these sweets, and eat a piece of fruit instead.

Fried Foods

With a stretch of fast food restaurants in every town in the country, it is easy to see why the population consumes so many fried foods. Fast food has quickly become a cheap alternative to cooking every night. With the majority of adults working full time, picking up a quick bite to eat for dinner seems like a no-brainer. It's true when they say you get what you pay for. Fast food contains very little fiber and a huge amount of carbs, making it hard to digest. These types of foods are typically high in calories with little to no nutritional value. If you combine the habit of eating fast food several times a week with a fairly sedentary lifestyle, you run the risk of gaining weight and all of the health problems that come with it. The majorities of fried foods start out as frozen and highly processed. This means that they contain a large amount of saturated fat. Even some of the healthy options listed on the menu, such as salads, could have upwards of 2000 calories. 2000 calories are the daily caloric intake for some people. You have to watch out for unhealthy add-ons such as dressings, crotons, and fried onions.

White Flour and White Rice

The white flour is in almost all of the foods listed above. White flour, rice, and other refined grains have been highly processed. Manufactures strip these foods of their brown coating which removes the majority of the fiber content along with it. Your body digests these refined ingredients very quickly causing you to feel sleepy and unmotivated. White carbs have been refined, which basically means that have been processed and have traded the majority of their fiber content for sugary carbs. This causes them to be digested rapidly by the body and stored as fat. Trade your white carbs for whole grain options such as whole wheat bread, brown rice, or quinoa. Cutting out white carbs is a great way to cut fat from your middle.

Refined Sweeteners and Sugars

Refined sugars and sweeteners increase insulin levels in the body. When your insulin levels increase, they promote the storage of fat. You can find refined sweeteners and sugars in almost all packaged food, and maybe even in your pantry. That's right, even white sugar that we use to cook with is bad for you! High fructose corn syrup is another culprit that will help pile on those pounds. Healthier alternatives include small amounts of maple sugar and real honey.

Fruit Juices

People tend to be unable to differentiate between calories they eat and calories they drink, and most people have been taught that fruit juice is good for them when it actually isn't. Fruit juice is filled with (you guessed it) sugar, and we all know that excess sugar is stored as fat within out fat cells, especially the ones in your belly.

Potatoes

Did you know that eating a baked potato does the same thing to your body as eating a tablespoon of sugar? Potatoes are filled with empty calories and are digested quickly. This means that you will be hungry and ready for more food long before you should be!

Pizza

Even though everyone in the world loves pizza, you have to ask yourself what is in pizza. The answer: Processed, refined crust topped with processed meats, filled with empty calories and a sprinkle of high-fat lactose on top. Pizza is filled with saturated fat, carbs, and sodium. Do not worry; you won't have to give up pizza forever. There are countless healthy alternatives to traditional pizza that are just as delicious.

Wisdom to Consider

Do not let this long list of no-no's get you down. It is important to consider your eating habits in order to change them. Pay attention to how, and what you eat throughout the day and monitor what you crave. Learn how to identify triggers that make you want to snack, either from stress or from boredom. You could spend a day writing down your eating habits to track areas of improvement.

When faced with making a lifestyle change, such as eating clean, try to reword your thoughts. Do not think of food as good or bad. Ask yourself if your food choice will help your goal or hurt your goal, but do not try to be a perfectionist. Remember that Rome was not built in a day, and neither is a healthier lifestyle. Do not beat yourself up for slipping. Take the opportunity to learn from it and continue down your path to a flat belly. If you expect too much from yourself, you will most likely crash and burn out before you even get started.

Finally, plan for your meals. Try to avoid situations where you aren't sure where your next meal will come from. This causes a sense of uncertainty that makes it really easy to choose something bad for you out of "necessity". Meal prepping is a great way to avoid this issue. You may even find that you enjoy cooking yummy, nutritional food once you get the hang of it!

Chapter 6: Healthy Diet

Diets to Consider

The key to eating a healthy diet is understanding how different foods affect the body. Now that you are aware of how the food you eat is processed into energy or fat and how processed foods negatively impact you, you can begin exploring healthier options. Choose foods that you enjoy and food that make you feel good. There are several diets out there that incorporate nutritious foods in a straightforward fashion. These diets include the Adkins Diet, which is a low carb, rapid weight loss diet, and the Paleo diet, which focuses on whole, unprocessed foods. Some people think of eating a healthy diet as a difficult task, but the best way to see it is as a creative opportunity for a skinnier, healthier you!

Foods to Eat

You may have already gathered this from the information above, but choosing whole foods that have not been processed is the best course of action. Watch out for things that come in packaging, even if the package says that the product is diet friendly. Getting all of the nutrients that you need is also important. The list below expands on the food you should eat to hold onto that sexy figure!

- **Plant oils** – olive oil, avocado oil, coconut oil, and other plant oils
- **Dairy products** – cottage cheese, Greek yogurt, and milk
- **Lean meats** – poultry and fish
- **Whole grains** – whole wheat, brown rice, steel cut oats, and quinoa

- **Whole fruit** – apples, oranges, bananas, grapefruit, and any other whole fruit you enjoy
- **Nuts** – walnuts, cashews, almonds, and pecans
- **Seeds** –sunflower, hemp, chia, and pumpkin seeds
- **Beans** – chickpeas, black beans, red beans, lentils, and kidney beans
- **Vegetables** – Carrots, cucumbers, avocado, tomato, celery, squash, spinach, kale, peas, onions, Brussels sprouts, sweet potatoes, corn, and bell peppers.

How Much You Should Eat

Once you have determined your daily caloric intake, it is time to think about how much you should eat, and what that should consist of. Sticking to the food groups mentioned above is the first step to your daily meals, but how much of each category should you consume in a 24-hour span? You want to be full after you eat but not stuffed, and you do not want to be left hungry. The balance lies somewhere in the middle. A good rule of thumb is to section your plate into three sections. The biggest section should be reserved for vegetables. Fresh veggies should make up the largest percent of your meals. The second largest section should be whole grains and healthy proteins. The smallest section of your plate should be fruits. When cooking a meal, think about how it will look on your plate. In order to look pretty, you must eat pretty. You should aim for colorful meals that provide lots of vitamins and minerals. Try to avoid large amounts of salt and sugar and enjoy the natural flavors of a wholesome, healthy diet.

Avoiding Overeating

The most significant thing to keep in mind when eating healthy is to strategize so that you do not overeat. To avoid overeating, choose smaller portions and chew slowly. Be mindful of how your body feels when you are eating so that when you are full, you know when to stop. Eliminate distractions such as TV and social media during mealtimes to help with mindful eating.

Eat and prepare your meals at home. This goes back to planning out your meal so that you do not end up stuck without a healthy option. Fast food and restaurants tend to give bigger portions and more calories than what we would prepare for ourselves at home.

Eat breakfast even if you do not want to. Skipping breakfast has gotten the reputation of being a good way to cut calories, but this is not the case. Having a healthy breakfast is the best way to level your blood sugar and kick-start your metabolism. Not to mention, when you do not eat breakfast, you are even hungrier by the middle of the day, which will lead to overeating.

Healthy Eating Mindset

Instead of only focusing on the food that you are and are not supposed to eat, focus on the reason why you want to lose weight. Develop a mantra that details your decision to become a healthier, thinner you and incorporate that thought into building your healthy habits. Be compassionate and kind to yourself, even when you do not feel like you've done a great job. Negativity will lead to throwing up your hands and giving in to the forbidden goodness of carbs and sugar. Tell yourself that you want to eat healthy, not that you have to eat healthy. Make the decision to think about the desire to choose healthy ingredients because of the way they make you feel.

Trust your body and pay attention to what it is telling you. Are you reaching for the Cheetos when you really want to rest? Are you craving that chocolate brownie when you actually want love and affection? As you incorporate healthy habits, teach yourself to slow down and breathe. Once you take the time to pause and question these bodily signals, you will begin to find the real meaning behind them. This opens up the door to fully understanding the best way to combat your cravings and triggers.

Be patient. Putting a time restriction on your weight loss goals will only make it that much more difficult to achieve. Setting a long-term goal and circling it in red on the calendar is counter-productive. Take every day as an opportunity to be better and do better, and see each daily success as something to be proud of. Trying to control every aspect of your lifestyle shift is only creating a trap for failure. You did not gain all of your weight in a week and you will not lose all of your weight in a week. Do not put unnecessary pressure on yourself by developing a strict lifestyle that is only going to bore you and tempt you to stray. Be understanding and more importantly, go with the flow.

Chapter 7: Meal Prep

Baked Honey-Mustard Chicken

Ingredients:
- 1 tsp. dried basil
- 1/2 c. honey
- 1/2 c. prepared mustard
- pepper and salt to taste
- 1 tsp. paprika
- 1/2 tsp. dried parsley
- 6 skinless, boneless chicken breast halves

How to prepare:
1. Preheat the oven to 175 degrees C (350 degrees F).
2. Rub salt and pepper on the chicken breasts and place in a 9x13-inch baking dish that's been greased lightly.
3. Mix together the parsley, paprika, basil, mustard, and honey, until well combined. 1/2 of this mixture should be poured and brushed over the chicken.
4. Bake the coated chicken breasts for 30 minutes in the oven. Flip the chicken when golden and with the remaining half of the honey mustard mixture, brush the chicken again.
5. Continue baking until the chicken is golden and cooked through.
6. Let cool 10 minutes before serving.

Slow Cooker Pork Tenderloin

Ingredients:

- black pepper (freshly ground) to taste
- 3 tbsp. soy sauce
- 3 tbsp. garlic (minced)
- 3/4 c. red wine
- 1 c. water
- 1 2 lbs. pork tenderloin
- 1 1 oz. envelope dry onion soup mix

How to prepare:

1. With the onion soup mix, place the pork in the slow cooker.
2. Pour the soy sauce, water, and wine on top. Flip the pork several times to ensure it is properly coated.
3. Gently spread garlic on the pork, try to leave it mostly on the top.
4. Add the pepper. Cook it covered for 4 hours on low.
5. Add drippings when you serve.

Roasted Vegetables

Ingredients:

- 1 small butternut squash
- 2 red bell peppers
- 1 sweet potato
- 1 tbsp. chopped fresh thyme
- black pepper (freshly ground) and salt to taste
- 3 Yukon Gold potatoes
- 1/4 c. olive oil
- 2 tbsp. fresh rosemary (chopped)
- 1 red onion
- 2 tbsp. balsamic vinegar

How to prepare:

1. Preheat the oven to 245 degrees C (475 degrees F)
2. Peel, cube, and dice the vegetables.
3. Combine the red bell peppers, Yukon potatoes, squash, red bell peppers sweet, and potato. Add the red onion to the mixture, breaking its layers off into pieces.
4. Stir the vinegar, rosemary, salt, pepper, and thyme together in a small bowl. Toss veggies until they are coated with the mixture. Then, on a roasting pan, spread them evenly.
5. Roast the vegetables for 35 to 40 minutes in the oven, stirring every few minutes until browned and cooked.

Fish Tacos

Ingredients:

- 1 egg
- 1 c. beer
- 1 tsp. baking powder
- 1/2 tsp. salt
- 2 tbsp. cornstarch
- 1 c. all-purpose flour
- 1 lime (juiced)
- 1/2 tsp. cumin (ground)
- 1 jalapeno pepper (minced)
- 1/2 c. mayonnaise
- 1-quart oil for frying
- 1/2 c. plain yogurt
- 1/2 tsp. oregano (dried)
- 1 tsp. capers (minced)
- 1/2 tsp. dill weed (dried)
- 1 tsp. cayenne pepper (ground)
- 1/2 medium cabbage (shredded)
- 1 12 oz. package corn tortillas
- 1 lb. cod fillets, sliced into portions of 2 to 3 oz.

How to prepare:

Beer Batter:

1. Mix the cornstarch, baking powder, salt, and flour together, then add the beer, egg. Add the flour into the mixture, stirring quickly, a few lumps are okay.

White Sauce:

1. Mix the mayonnaise and yogurt together. Gradually add in the lime juice— the consistency will be a bit runny.

Mix in dill, jalapeno, capers, oregano, cayenne, and cumin.
2. In deep-fryer, heat the oil to 190 degrees C (375 degrees F).
3. Lightly bread the fish pieces with flour. Dip it one by one into the batter, and cook until golden and crisp. Drain the fillets on paper towels.
4. Fry tortillas lightly, avoid getting them crisp.
5. In a tortilla, add shredded cabbage and then place the fish on top. Drizzle with white sauce.

Lentil Soup

Ingredients:

- 2 carrots (diced)
- 2 c. dry lentils
- 2 stalks celery (chopped)
- 1/4 c. olive oil
- 2 cloves garlic (minced)
- 1 14.5 oz. can crushed tomatoes
- 1 tsp. oregano (dried)
- 2 tbsp. vinegar
- 1 onion (chopped)
- 1 bay leaf
- 1 tsp. basil (dried)
- 8 c. water
- 1/2 c. spinach (sliced thinly)
- black pepper and salt to taste

How to prepare:

1. Heat oil on the stove, in medium heat. Mix in celery, carrots, and onions. Cook until onions are translucent.
2. Sauté in oregano, garlic, basil, and bay leaf for a few minutes.
3. Mix in the lentils, and then add tomatoes and water. Let it boil.
4. Let it simmer on low for at least an hour.
5. Add the spinach, just enough for it to wilt, then serve immediately.
6. Stir in the pepper, vinegar, and salt according to your taste, and more or less vinegar if desired.

Turkey Veggie Meatloaf Cups

Ingredients:

- 1 lb. extra lean turkey (ground)
- 1 red bell pepper (chopped)
- 1 egg
- 2 c. zucchini (chopped)
- 1/2 c. uncooked couscous
- 1 1/2 c. onions (chopped)
- 1/2 c. barbecue sauce, or as needed
- 2 tbsp. Worcestershire sauce
- 1 tbsp. Dijon mustard

How to prepare:

1. Preheat oven to 200 degrees C (400 degrees F)
2. Using a cooking spray, grease 20 muffin cups.
3. In a food processor, add zucchini, red bell pepper, and onions. Process until finely chopped, and NOT liquefied. Place the mixture in a bowl and add in couscous, egg, Worcestershire sauce, ground turkey, and Dijon mustard. Mix until properly incorporated.
4. Spoon the meatloaf mixture into each muffin cup, filling it by about 3/4. Smear a teaspoon of barbecue sauce at the top.
5. Bake for about 20 minutes or until the juices run clear.
6. let it cool for 5 minutes before serving.

Grandma's Chicken Noodle Soup

Ingredients:

- 2 1/2 c. wide egg noodles
- 3 c. cooked chicken meat (diced)
- 12 c. chicken broth
- 1 tsp. vegetable oil
- 1 tsp. poultry seasoning
- 1 1/2 tbsp. salt
- 1/4 c. water
- 1 c. celery (chopped)
- 1 c. onion (chopped)
- 1/3 c. cornstarch

How to prepare:

1. Prepare a pot of lightly salted water; let it boil over the stovetop.
2. Add the oil and egg noodles. Let it cook until tender. Drain and rinse under cool running water.
3. Mix salt, poultry seasoning, and broth in a large saucepan. Allow to boil. Add in onion and celery. Cover and let it simmer on low for 15 minutes.
4. Mix water and cornstarch together in a small bowl, until cornstarch is completely dissolved.
5. While stirring the soup constantly, add the cornstarch mix. Add the chicken and noodles. Cook until heated through.

Chicken and Asparagus Pasta

Ingredients:

- 1 package 16 oz. penne pasta
- 2 chicken breast halves, skinless and boneless (cubed)
- 1 clove garlic (thinly sliced)
- 1 bunch slender asparagus spears (sliced diagonally)
- 5 tbsp. olive oil (divided)
- 1/4 c. Parmesan cheese
- 1/2 c. low-sodium chicken broth
- Pepper, garlic powder, and salt to taste

How to prepare:

1. Prepare a large pot of lightly salted water; bring it to a boil over the stovetop.
2. Add in the penne and cook until tender, but also firm to the bite (about 5 to 8 minutes). Drain, and set aside.
3. In a large skillet, heat 3 tablespoons olive oil over medium-high heat. Add in chicken. Season with pepper, garlic powder, and salt. Cook until chicken is golden and cooked through. Set aside, drain oil on paper towels.
4. Add in the chicken broth into the skillet. Mix in garlic, asparagus, salt, pepper, and garlic powder. Put the lid on and cook until the asparagus is just tender, about 6 to 8 minutes. Add the chicken back into the skillet. Cook until heated through.
5. Combine the sauce and the pasta. Let it cool for 5 minutes before serving. Stir in 2 tablespoons of olive oil, and then top with Parmesan cheese.

Greek Chicken Pasta

Ingredients:

- 1 lb. chicken breast, skinless and boneless (cubed)
- 1/2 c. red onion (chopped)
- 1 can 14 oz. marinated artichoke hearts (drained and chopped)
- 1 package 16 oz. linguine pasta
- 1 tbsp. olive oil
- 2 cloves garlic (crushed)
- 2 lemons for garnish (wedged)
- 2 tbsp. lemon juice
- 1 large tomato (chopped)
- 2 tsp. oregano (dried)
- 1/2 c. feta cheese (crumbled)
- 3 tbsp. fresh parsley (chopped)
- pepper and salt to taste

How to prepare:

1. Prepare a large pot of lightly salted water; bring it to a boil over the stovetop.
2. Add in the penne and cook until tender, but also firm to the bite (about 5 to 8 minutes). Drain, and set aside.
3. In a large skillet, heat olive oil on medium-high heat. Sauté garlic and onion until fragrant. Add in the chicken, cook until the juices run clear and chicken is cooked through and golden.
4. Reduce heat to medium-low. Mix in cooked pasta, artichoke hearts, tomato, oregano, lemon juice, parsley, and feta cheese. Cook until heated through.
5. Remove from heat, season with pepper and salt. Garnish with lemon wedges.

Black Bean Chili

Ingredients:

- 1 lb. turkey (ground)
- 1 onion (diced)
- 1 tbsp. vegetable oil
- 1 14.5 oz. can crushed tomatoes
- 3 15 oz. cans black beans (do not drain)
- 2 cloves garlic (minced)
- 1 1/2 tbsp. chili powder
- 1 tbsp. oregano (dried)
- 1 tbsp. basil leaves (dried)
- 1 tbsp. red wine vinegar

How to prepare:

1. In a large pot, heat the oil over medium heat.
2. Sauté garlic and onion, cook until onions are translucent.
3. Add the turkey, sauté until cooked through and golden.
4. Mix in tomatoes, beans, oregano, chili powder, vinegar, and basil.
5. Put the lid over it and simmer on low for 1 hour or more, until flavors are well blended.

Feta and Spinach Pita Bake

Ingredients:

- 4 fresh mushrooms (sliced)
- 6 6-inch whole wheat pita bread
- 2 Roma (plum) tomatoes (chopped)
- 1 6 oz. tub sun-dried tomato pesto
- 1 bunch spinach (chopped)
- 2 tbsp. Parmesan cheese (grated)
- 3 tbsp. olive oil
- 1/2 c. feta cheese (crumbled)
- ground black pepper to taste

How to prepare:

1. Preheat the oven to 175 degrees C (350 degrees F).
2. Brush tomato pesto on one side of each pita bread. Place them on a baking sheet, pesto-side up.
3. Top pitas with mushrooms, spinach, tomatoes, Parmesan cheese, and feta cheese. Drizzle with olive oil and sprinkle with pepper.
4. Bake in the oven until pita bread is crisp. Slice into quarters.

Zucchini and Potato Bake

Ingredients:

- 4 medium potatoes, (peeled and sliced into large chunks)
- 2 medium zucchini (sliced into large pieces)
- 1 medium red bell pepper (chopped)
- 1 clove garlic (sliced)
- 1/2 c. dry bread crumbs
- 1/4 c. olive oil
- ground black pepper and salt to taste
- paprika to taste

How to prepare:

1. Preheat oven to 200 degrees C (400 degrees F).
2. Combine the potatoes, red bell pepper, zucchini, bread crumbs, olive oil, and garlic. Season with pepper, salt, and paprika.
3. Bake it in the oven for an hour. Mixing occasionally until potatoes are lightly brown and tender.

Quinoa Tabbouleh

Ingredients:

- 2 c. water
- 1 c. quinoa
- 2 carrots (grated)
- 1 cucumber (diced)
- 3 tomatoes (diced)
- 1 c. fresh parsley (chopped)
- 2 bunches green onions (diced)
- 1/4 c. olive oil
- 1/2 tsp. sea salt
- 1/4 c. lemon juice
- 1 pinch salt

How to prepare:

1. In a saucepan, bring water to a boil. Add a pinch of salt and the quinoa. Switch heat to low, put a lid over it, and allow to simmer for 15 minutes. Let it cool, and then fluff it with a fork.
2. Combine sea salt, olive oil, cucumber, tomatoes, lemon juice, green onions, parsley, and carrots in a large bowl. Stir in cooled quinoa.

Chapter 8: What to Drink

How Can Beverages Help You Lose Weight?

Eating healthy and exercising are the two most essential aspects of getting a flat belly, but you can give them an extra push by pairing them with healthy drinking habits. Some beverages come with a multitude of health benefits that can make you feel and look like a whole new person. None of the drinks listed below are processed or high in sugar. As always, the most natural approach is the most beneficial when it comes to your fitness goals. Whether the drinks boosts your metabolism or allow you to shed water weight, you should consider adding them to your new lifestyle!

Water

Water may be the most important beverage to consume, not only when you are attaining the perfect body, but all the time. Water helps your body function properly by hydrating your organs on a molecular level. Without water, your body does not function properly. Being dehydrated can cause your body to become stressed and affect how much fat you are burning by slowing down your metabolism to save energy. Water is also a natural appetite suppressant. As you know, when the stomach feels full, it sends messages to your brain telling it that you are not hungry.

When you drink water, it takes up space in your belly causing you to feel full with literally none of the calories. Sometimes, your body may tell you that you are hungry when you are actually thirsty. If you are feeling hungry right after a meal, or when you know that you shouldn't be starving, drinking water should take care of it.

As previously mentioned, water can help your body burn calories by boosting your metabolism. One study shows individuals who drank 500 mL of room temperature or cold water burned 3% more calories than they usually would 2 hours after they drank the water. This is especially true if you drink ice water since your body burns calories to heat the water up to body temperature.

Staying hydrated ensures that your body can effectively remove waste. Water allows your kidneys to flush out toxins while holding onto electrolytes and nutrients. If the body is dehydrated then the kidneys retain fluid in attempts to rehydrate. When you do not have enough water, you could become constipated which causes you to feel bloated and full. This can add anywhere from an inch to three inches to your waist. Drinking plenty of water can allow you to avoid retaining waist and adding extra pounds to your middle.

Green Tea

Green tea has become highly popular in the health community over the past several years, and for good reason. This miracle drink contains a high number of antioxidants known as catechins. Catechins have been known to quickly rehydrate the body while burning stubborn belly fat. They do this by increasing the release of fat from fat cells while also increasing your liver's fat burning potential. Green tea also has anti-inflammatory properties. If ingested regularly, it can offset inflammation in the belly and stop slow weight gain. Several studies have concluded that drinking green tea on a regular basis can help shrink your middle and boost your immune system.

Apple Cider Vinegar

Even though it smells less than appetizing, apple cider vinegar (ACV) is actually known for its ability to aid in weight loss and fitness goals. ACV acts as a bile stimulant and allows the pH level in the lining of your stomach to balance. This unorthodox beverage can suppress your appetite and aid in the removal of waste from your body. Try mixing warm water with a spoon full of apple cider vinegar and drinking it first thing in the morning, on an empty stomach to see the amazing effects.

Peppermint Tea

Peppermint tea is not only a refreshing summertime beverage but also a handy tool used to aid in weight loss. Drinking peppermint tea ensures that your body is digesting food quickly and efficiently. It helps to relieve bloating which is linked to fat accumulation in the abdominal area. Bloating could be caused by food not being digested properly, which peppermint tea prevents. Peppermint tea also prevents and reduces heartburn, aids in restful sleep, and keeps your skin looking and feeling amazing. Try incorporating peppermint tea into your routine to give your overall wellness a boost!

Cinnamon

As you know, eating spicy foods can increase your metabolism because they cause your body temperature to increase. This process is called thermogenesis, which is how your cells create energy from the food we eat and turn it into heat. The same thing happens when you ingest cinnamon. The antioxidants in this miracle spice have anti-inflammatory properties, which help to reduce belly fat in the form of bloating and constipation. You can add cinnamon to a bottle of water to make it more appetizing or you could have it with your morning coffee. Either way, cinnamon is a tasty way to keep your diet on track for the perfect flat belly.

Coffee

Some of you may be relieved to find this morning staple on the list. If you can't function without your cup of joe first thing in the morning, then you're in luck. Black coffee has been known to supply a long list of health benefits that stem from its caffeine content. These health benefits include aiding in weight loss by converting fat into energy. If you are looking to switch it up, green coffee has been known to increase fat loss even more so than its darker sibling. Green coffee is coffee beans that haven't been roasted. Green coffee is particularly high in chlorogenic acid, which has been proven to ramp up your metabolism, and treats your body to a healthy dose of antioxidants. The trick to allowing coffee to help your diet is to keep sugar and creamer out of it. Although tasty, this add-in is high in calories and fat, which directly influence the coffee's ability to reduce fat from your middle.

Chapter 9: Working with Your Metabolism

What is Metabolism?

The dictionary definition of metabolism is the chemical process that occurs within all living organisms in order to maintain life. In other words, metabolism if how our bodies convert the food we eat into energy. During this biochemical process, calories are combined with oxygen in order to release the energy we need to carry out our everyday lives. There are two separate functions of metabolism: catabolism and anabolism. Catabolism is defined as the release of energy from calories and anabolism is defined as the creation and storage of energy from calories. All aspects of metabolism are controlled by the endocrine system, which is in charge of countless bodily functions such as mood regulation, reproductive functions, and cell tissue growth. Even though it is not possible to completely control your metabolism, it is possible to influence it using three key methods: the food you eat, the quantity of food you eat, and how much exercise you get every day.

We all know someone who seems to be able to eat whatever they want and never gain a pound. We usually chalk this up to their fast metabolism and envy them for being so lucky, but having a fast metabolism is actually just a myth. Your age, gender, diet, activity levels, and genetics determine your metabolic rate. The chances of all of these aspects aligning perfectly to give someone an effort-free, perfect body is unrealistic. The secret to their success has nothing to do with their luck and everything to do with their balance. People who seem to have a fast metabolism are probably already skinny, highly active, and get plenty of restful sleep every night. Like most things, there is no magic solution to a metabolism that will benefit you. It takes attentiveness and dedication to train your metabolism to adhere to your needs and not work against you. Do not be discouraged. With practice and trial and error, you could double your metabolic rate in no time. A huge advantage to understanding your metabolism is that changing it seems much more attainable.

Age and Metabolism

You may have heard people talk about how they are not able to eat like their younger selves. You may have even had someone tell you that your eating habits will catch up to your metabolism. Unfortunately, age does play a large role in metabolic rate. As you grow older, your metabolism slows down. This makes it easier to gain weight and difficult to lose it. Physical activity tends to slow as you age, so the amount of energy you burn decreases. When your activity levels lower so does your muscle mass, causing your body to need even fewer calories for energy. Even though you can become less active and slower to burn calories when you age, there are several steps you can take to boost your metabolism and get that flat belly.

Eating to Boost Your Metabolism

Most diets require you to count calories and keep track of how many you are eating in a day. With metabolism, it isn't about how much you eat, but what you are eating. Simply eating breakfast can increase your metabolism for a short amount of time. This is because of the thermic effect of food (TEF), which is caused by the extra energy needed to absorb, digest, and process the nutrients in your food. The best way to fully take advantage of this process is by eating plenty of protein. This is because protein causes the biggest rise in TEF. Having a healthy dose of protein in your meal can increase your metabolic rate upwards of 15%. When you compare this to 2% for fats and 7% for carbs, there is no doubt that protein is the superhero of a strong metabolism. Studies show that individuals eat 440 fewer calories a day when 30% of their diet was made up of protein. This is because protein keeps you fuller longer, making it easier to maintain your caloric deficit. Consuming a large amount of lean meat and plant protein allows your body to combat muscle loss. So, getting enough protein is key for anyone who is undergoing a large reduction in fat, such as yourself!

Protein isn't the only food to keep in mind when boosting your metabolism; spicy foods can also increase your ability to burn fat. Spicy food such as peppers contains a substance known as capsaicin. Capsaicin is the compound used to produce the burning sensation caused by consuming spice. Even though capsaicin is a biological sign to deter mammals, including humans, it is great at increasing resting metabolic rate. Studies show that eating peppers in bearable doses can result in the body burning up to 10 extra calories per meal. Even though you cannot rely on spicy food alone to lose weight, combined with other metabolism boosting practices is can provide a weight loss advantage.

While you are in the process of adding protein-rich foods and peppers to your diet, consider how many times a day you would like to eat. The tradition three meals a day could be holding back your metabolic potential. When you eat large amounts with a big span of time in between, your metabolism slows down to preserve your energy. Eating a snack or a small meal every 3 to 4 hours will allow your metabolism to streamline and burn more calories than it would if you only eat at breakfast, lunch, and dinner. Studies show that people who snack often feel less hungry and eat less at meal times. Eating more frequently tends to have a positive impact on more than just cutting calories. Healthy snacking can actually stabilize blood glucose levels. Smaller meals have less glucose than their larger counterparts. This causes your blood sugar to rise at a much slower rate, keeping cortisol levels low and hunger at bay. This type of diet is especially beneficial for those who suffer from diabetes or hypoglycemia. It is import to remember to eat healthy snacks, even if they are small.

Drinking to Boost Your Metabolism

Food is not the only thing in your toolbox that can influence your metabolism! We have discussed the importance of cutting sugary beverages from your diet because of the excess calories. These empty calories also affect your metabolic rate simply by increasing the number of calories you are consuming as a whole. The straightforward solution is to drink water. Water has no calories and keeps your body hydrated. In fact, drinking water speeds up metabolism temporarily and even more so if the water you are drinking is ice cold. Research suggests that drinking a half-liter of water can increase your resting metabolic rate by upwards of 20% for approximately an hour. Your body will need even more energy to heat the water up to body temperature, giving you an extra fat burning boost. Try drinking a glass of water before your next meal to keep you from feeling hungry. Studies prove that overweight individuals who drank water before sitting down to a meal lost 40% more weight than individuals who didn't. Think of water as your secret weapon to a slim waist.

Even though drinking water is essential for a flat belly, there are two other solutions to hydrating yourself and boosting metabolism. The first of the two would be drinking green tea. Green tea is low in calories. So, drinking this tea is good for weight loss and weight maintenance. Green tea has been known to convert excess fat stored in the body to free fatty acids. This increases your fat burning potential to upwards of 15%. It can actually increase your metabolic rate by 5%. Green tea is a great way to mix up your beverage routine. Add a small amount of real, organic honey to curve your sweet tooth and boost your metabolism at the same time.

Coffee is the second solutions to your worn out water routine. Most of us can't live without coffee regardless, but did you know that it could actually boost your metabolism while it gives you the extra kick to start your morning. The secret to this miracle liquid is caffeine. The caffeine in black coffee can actually increase your ability to burn fat by 10%. The more weight you lose, the more fat you can burn by drinking coffee. Research suggests that lean people who drank coffee increased their metabolism double that of an obese person. Talk about the drink that keeps on giving!

Sleep and Metabolism

The same way that stress can affect your weight loss goal, so can your sleeping habits. When your body is sleep deprived, it increases the level of cortisol. This sends hunger signals to your brain, which in turn causes you to crave comfort foods such as carbs and fats. Lack of sleep has been linked to a huge increase in obesity in America. Kicking cravings into high gear isn't the only set back of a sleepless night. When your body is tired, your blood sugar levels and insulin resistance skyrockets, which puts the body at a higher risk or developing diabetes. The most important thing to remember is to go to bed. Get plenty of rest so that your body is in tiptop shape to shed pounds and flatten your middle. Unfortunately, getting 8 hours of sleep every night isn't always realistic. The next time you suffer from a less than restful night, remember that your body is under stress and will want to consume tenfold to make up for the trauma.

Exercise and Metabolism

You should think of your flat belly journey as a two-sided scale (pardon the pun). On one side you have your diet, and on the other side, you have your exercise routine. It takes a calculated amount on both sides to garner success. When thinking about influencing your metabolism, you should use the same concept. Increasing your metabolism with physical activity can be as simple as standing up more. That's right! Something as simple as investing in a standing desk or taking short walking breaks during your working hours can burn an extra 175 calories a day!

When it comes to increasing your metabolism, you will want to do more than just stand up. Muscle cells require an exponential amount of energy, which means the more muscle you have, the more calories you burn even while you are at rest. The best way to gain muscle mass, even when dieting, is by lifting heavy things. The human body is very adaptive, so when you lift heavy weight on a regular basis your muscles grow to accommodate the weight. Increasing the pounds you lift will cause your muscle mass to grow and your metabolism to increase, as well. So, take every opportunity to bench, squat, deadlift, and row to see less flab and more fab!

Once you have mastered the art of heavy lifting, pair it with High-Intensity Interval Training (HIIT) to take full advantage of how exercise can increase your metabolism. HIIT is a system of exercise that pushes your body to the limit and then allows it to rest, only to start the process back over again. Similar to lifting weights, this type of exercise allows you to burn more fat by increasing your heart rate and allowing your body to adapt to the level of activity over time. This is why running for short periods of time has proven to be better for metabolism than jogging for long periods of time. In fact, any intense exercise that you do can be done in a fraction of the time with better results. For example, if you do 1 full minute of squats and 1 minute of rest over and over again, you will see more results than if you do 3 sets of 10 squats over the course of 20 minutes because of the way your heart beat increases. So, not only will HIIT exercises save you time, but it will also give you better results. This is true regardless of age.

Chapter 10: Cardio and Strength Training

Understanding Exercise

Staying physically active is essential to achieving a flat belly and maintaining your overall health. Exercise is an activity that requires physical effort, with the purpose of improving or sustaining health and fitness. Exercising can help decrease your risk of serious diseases such as obesity, osteoporosis, heart disease, and some cancer. It also is beneficial to your mental health, helping you to release tension and relax. To lose weight you have to burn more calories than you consume. You can do this by eating a healthy diet and exercising regularly. Two of the best exercises to perform to help you get a flat belly are aerobic exercises and strength training. Combine these with a low caloric intake and you will have the body of your dreams before you know it!

Aerobic Exercise

Aerobic exercises are any various sustained exercises just like jogging, cycling running, swimming, or rowing, that stimulates and strengthens the lungs and heart, and at the same time improve the body's oxygen utilization. In layman's terms, Aerobic exercise is cardio. Studies show that cardio is one of the most effective exercises to eliminate belly fat. It is important to keep in mind that the frequency of your cardio is more important than the intensity. Research suggests that people lost more fat from all areas of their body when they performed aerobic exercise for 500 minutes a week compared to those who performed 300 minutes a week.

Cardio is all about losing weight and not about building muscle mass. There are plenty of sources out there that will try to convince you those 500 crunches a day or the latest and greatest abdominal machine will give you a flat belly, but that is not the case. To achieve a flat stomach you must remove the layer of fat that covers your abdominal muscles. Cardio is the only solution to shedding that extra layer and luckily, it is fantastic at burning calories! The trick to cardio is getting your blood pumping. Once you begin to move and get your heart rate into your target zone (how many beats per minute you need to burn calories) you will start to sweat and breathe harder. During this process, your body begins to burn calories. You burn more calories the harder and longer you work. It is important to find an aerobic exercise that you enjoy so that you do not feel like your fitness routine is a chore. Even going for a brisk walk every day will help you burn off the belly fat.

Strength Training

Regardless of which aerobic activity you choose, it is important to combine it with High-Intensity Interval Training (HIIT). This type of exercise gets your blood pumping while pushing your muscles to their limit. Lifting weights strengthen your bones and add muscle mass to your body. Having more muscle mass will allow you to burn more calories while you are at rest. Heavy lifting has also been known to increase energy levels as well as self-esteem. Even though strength training does not directly affect your abdomen, when fat within your muscles decrease, you will appear less flabby and more toned. Toning your muscles along with consistent cardio will improve your weight loss progress, but do not expect to see results by work on your abs alone.

It is important to focus on major muscles groups throughout the body in order to add more muscle mass. Important groups to focus on include your chest, back, hips, triceps, biceps, shoulders, buttocks, calves, thighs, and forearms. As you work to build these muscle groups, your body will need more calories causing your metabolism to reach its highest potential. This means that the majority of the healthy food you eat will go to feeding your growing muscles and not to your fat cells. Along with this, your conditioned heart will be even better at burning calories, giving you the perfect combination to shed those inches.

It is important to remember that as the fat falls off of your body, your belly will shrink too. You should think of fat as an organ that lies throughout the entire body. You can't remove fat from one part of your body at a time unless you use a medical procedure such as liposuction. As the percentage of fat lowers, you will see the changes everywhere, including your belly. That doesn't mean that you should not work your abs, even though you should be strategic about how you do it.

Always exercise your abs at the end of your work out. You want to do this because you are indirectly using them for all of the exercises you perform. Your abdominal muscles are considered stabilizer muscles that you should use to keep your form perfect while strength training for optimal results. If you focus on your middle muscles for the first step of your work out, they will be too tired to hold your form throughout the rest of your exercise regimen. Remember to work down from the biggest muscle groups, such as the legs, to the smallest muscle group, such as the abs.

Strengthening your core is essential to getting a flat belly. The tried and true method of crunches and sit-ups are effective in strengthening your core since they work the largest abdominal muscles that are in charge of flexing the spine. The same muscle group compresses the abdomen to provide a trim waist. This is not the only muscle group to watch out for. The internal and external obliques sit on the sides of the abdomen and hold everything together. You use these muscles when you bend sideways or twist at the spine. Working these muscles often is important since they also compress the abdomen. To get optimal results from working these muscles, try adding a twist to your crunches or even small dumbbells. The lower abs are located below the obliques at your sides. This is a problem area for most women, especially postpartum. In order to strengthen this muscle group, concentrate on lifting the lower body instead of the upper body with exercises such as leg raises.

What to Watch out For

It is a common assurance for you to be hungrier when you work out. It is true that you will need more calories after you have established your fitness routine. Some people find it easier to overestimate the number of calories they have burned, which then causes them to overeat. It is important to focus on healthy eating at this phase of your journey so that you can maintain your weight loss momentum. Some people become hungrier and want to eat even more, while others have a loss of appetite after exercise. This is known as "exercise anorexia" which is tied to a decrease in the hunger hormone ghrelin. The effect that exercise has on your appetite varies between individual.

Chapter 11: The Big Picture

Deciding to make a lifestyle change to become the person that you want to be is never easy. Especially when you are faced with challenges that you have never encountered before. Getting fit is a major decision, but one that will benefit you every day for the rest of your life. Now that you are equipped with the tools to begin your health and fitness journey, you will see the pounds begin to fall off. Do not be discouraged if your weight begins to plateau or it seems impossible to lose the last inch of flab left on your belly.

Working off the unwanted weight will not always be easy. In fact, there may be days where you want to throw up your hands, scream, and quit in frustration. It takes upwards of 6 weeks to truly reap the benefits of your new lifestyle. Until then, you will want to navigate your new habits with a positive mindset, reminding yourself that everyone struggles to adapt to a new routine at first. You will be sore, you will be tired, and you will most likely be a little hungry, but all of this will be worth it when you can look in the mirror and see the person you have always dreamed of being. On the days where you feel like giving in, remember to be grateful for the new person you are becoming and all of the hard work that you have completed. You will want to be grateful for your newfound energy and your growing confidence.

Now that you have made the commitment to work for your dream body, you should know that your flat belly is not a destination. Your fitness goal should be seen as a continuous journey that constantly challenges you to be better. Think of yourself as an active person, even if you are dreading your afternoon run. Make the decision to walk more than you drive.

Recruit a friend or find an individual that is on the same journey that you are. Sometimes it is easier to get up and go if you know someone is waiting for you.

Be kind to yourself. Remember that even Olympic athletes have rest days to let their bodies recover. Listen to your body and do not be afraid to take a day off from the gym or go super slow on your run. These things are an important part of getting a flat belly and reaching your fitness goals. If you overwork your body you could badly damage your muscles, making it even harder to get to where you want to be. Do not be frightened to change your routine as you grow and change. Nothing ever stays the same forever and neither should your wellness practices. Transition, although sometimes difficult, is a healthy part of physical and mental growth.

With the tools provided in the previous pages of this book, you have everything you need to eat clean, train hard, and turn heads wherever you go!

Conclusion

Thanks for making it through to the end of *How to Lose Belly Fat: A Complete Guide to Losing Weight and Achieving a Flat Belly*. Let's hope it was informative and able to provide you with all of the tools you need to achieve your fitness goals!

The next step is to put actions to words and work for the perfect flat belly!

BONUS:

As a way of saying thank you for purchasing my book, please use your link below to claim your 3 FREE Cookbooks on Health, Fitness & Dieting Instantly

https://bit.ly/2LEQVu2

You can also share your link with your friends and families whom you think that can benefit from the cookbooks or you can forward them the link as a gift!

Made in the USA
Coppell, TX
29 April 2021